HOW TO STAY HEALTHY During/After the COVID-19 Pandemic?

A HANDBOOK FOR SURVIVING

Keep your body immune strong as Superman!

JING CARTER-LU

PAGE PUBLISHING
Conneaut Lake, PA

First originally published by Page Publishing 2022

ISBN 978-1-6624-5927-6 (pbk)
ISBN 978-1-6624-5926-9 (digital)

Printed in the United States of America

CONTENTS

INTRODUCTION

Today is December 25, 2020, the Christmas holiday. I finally get a chance to take a break from my busy work schedules. I wake up in the morning and think through what I have done in 2020 and what happened in the world in the year 2020.

What really changed people's lives in the year 2020 was the COVID-19 pandemic situation. It caused many schools to close. It caused many stores, offices, and restaurants to close.

In 2020, people focused on fighting the COVID-19 disease and trying to stop it from spreading to more people. Sick people were isolated in hospitals for treatment. *Facemasks were a must to go into stores and meetings and six feet of social distance was required because the coronavirus was infectious and traveled through the air.*

I started to test many traditional methods that people used to stay healthy from cough and breathing problems to see if they can help with surviving during the COVID-19 pandemic. I was home-schooled for medicine since childhood because my father was a doctor and one of the managers who run a medicine and medical equipment company.

In 2020, I started to stay healthier with food medicine research, test some methods, and write a booklet titled *How to Stay Healthy During/After the COVID-19 Pandemic?*. It is focusing on some self-treatment to avoid getting sick from polluted air that might contain the COVID-19 virus. Then use food medicine to improve the immune system. And study on the human body's acupressure point (also called acupuncture point) that really worked to heal some pain symptoms and keep body strong.

The best of all is that these methods listed in this booklet do not cost much, and you can do it yourself to stay healthier.

I also provide a solution and focus on addressing an important issue—indoor air quality. So many people had to start working at home instead of going to offices because of the COVID-19 pandemic. Therefore, the indoor air quality at home becomes particularly important for people's health. All the air should be filtered before it blows into people's rooms. Here I introduce the product called Ceiling/Floor Vent's Eco Air Filters and its holder product to help you keep indoor air clean. It is made by Eco-safe Air Filter Manufacturing Company, which is based in the USA.

Filtering the air before it blows into each room in your house or apartment can help people stay healthier and avoid getting allergies and the COVID-19 virus. Use Ceiling/Floor Vent's Eco Air Filter to stop bugs from coming into rooms that can save people's lives in some cases.

CHAPTER 1

Keep Your Home Clean

The routine household cleaning work we usually do involves

a)   vacuuming the carpet area at least once per week,
b)   wiping down all furniture once a week, and
c)   mopping the floor as needed and with a weekly cleaning schedule.

If you have pets in your home, I suggest you do these two or three times per week and do it as needed to keep your home clean.

Mold Challenge

Molds grow and spread like pollen. Its spores float in the air, and we cannot see it with our naked eye because they are so tiny/little and lightweight. You might see it under the microscope in a research laboratory. They grow wherever they land on. We will see them when they grow bigger. At home, we do see mold continually coming back to our bathtub's edge, the bottom part of the shower curtain, and on the wall. That is why we must clean and brush the bathtub with bleach to remove the mold stains at least once per week.

There are three things that we can do to clean it out:

1. Brush it with liquid or powdered bleach cleaning products.

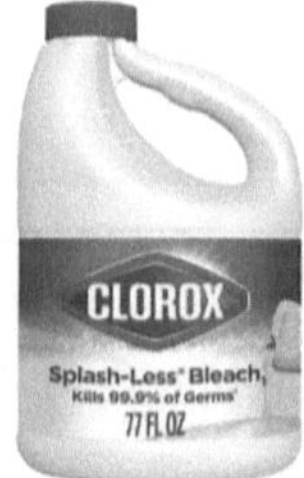
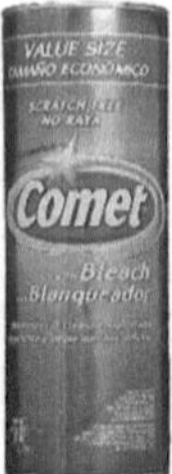

2. Spray the mold remover on the black/pink mold spots to remove it.

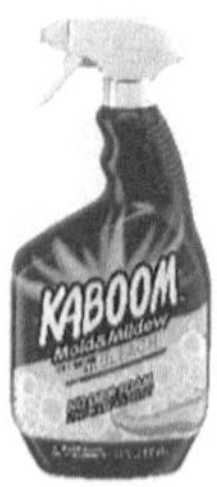

3. Use *Ceiling/Floor Vent's Eco Air Filter* to stop the mold from circulating in your home, especially in the bathroom.

Below are some pictures that demonstrated how Ceiling/Floor Vent's Eco Air Filters work:

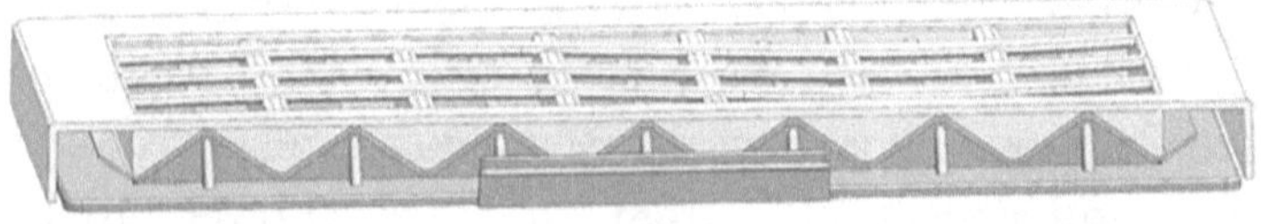

The pink color shown the FILTER SHEET in the Holder.

HOW TO STAY HEALTHY DURING/AFTER THE COVID-19 PANDEMIC?

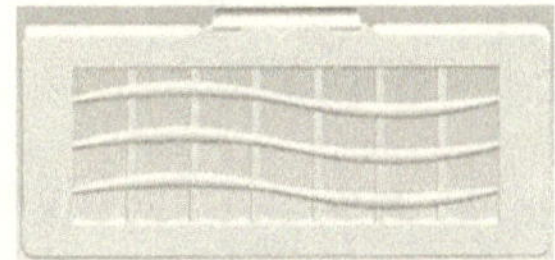

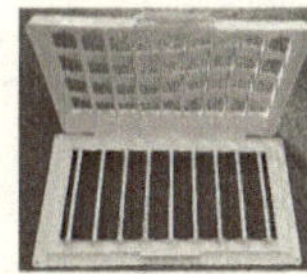

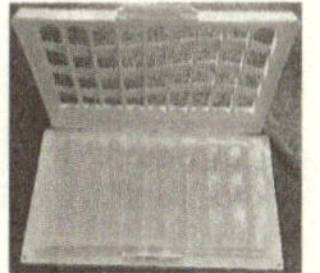

| Floor Vent's Air Filter Holder | Ceiling Vent's Air Filter Holder | Adding Eco Air Filter sheet |

(Opened the cap to add a filter sheet)

These unique products are created and manufactured by Eco-safe Air Filter Manufacturing Company in Georgia, USA.

They can customize the sizes of the sheets of the Eco Air Filters as per your request. Please send your purchase request by email to the Eco-safe Air Filter Manufacturing Company for help: sales@ EcosafeAirFilters.com.

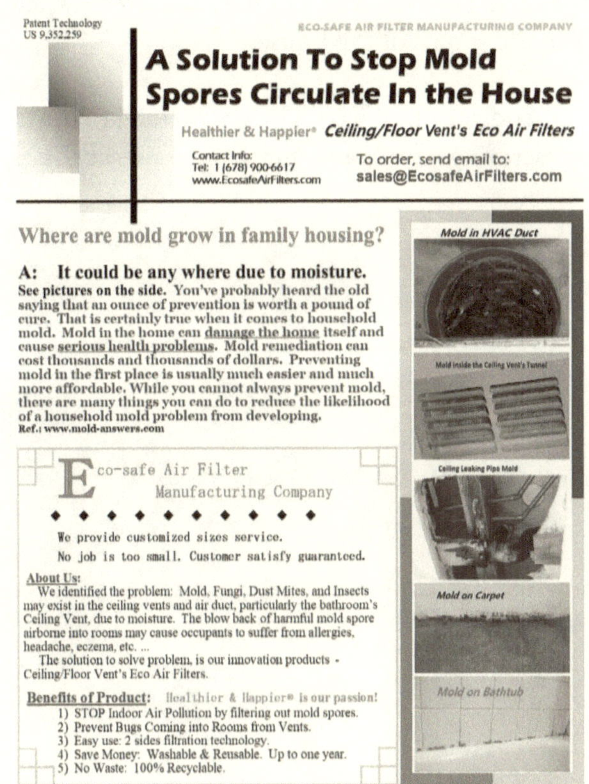

Bug Challenge

We all have experienced spiders, ants, roaches, etc. coming into our homes. We do not know how and where they come in. However, those bugs are in our environment.

What can we do to stop the bugs from coming into our homes?

a) Spray some cockroach killer in the corners of the kitchen floor and the area under the sink, where the bugs possibly hide.

b) In the closet or wherever you store clothes, use old-fashioned *mothballs*, which can kill clothes moths and their eggs and larvae.

c) Use *Ceiling/Floor Vent's Eco Air Filters* to stop the bugs, mold spores, and dust mites from coming inside through the ceiling or floor vents of the AC system, where air blows into the rooms of the house.

You can send your purchase request by email to the Eco-safe Air Filter Manufacturing Company for help: sales@EcosafeAirFilters.com.

Patent Technology
U.S. Patent# 9,352,259

A Solution To Prevent Bugs Come Into Room

We created the Ceiling / Wall / Floor Vent's Eco Air Filters to stop Bugs come into people's home to bite them. The solution is putting Vent's Eco Air Filters on all the Vents where air blows into rooms. It can STOP Bugs coming into rooms from the Vents.

Some Bugs bites are life-threatening! Some Bugs bites cause Allergies and diseases. Stop bugs coming into homes to save children's lives! (Ref. pictures: www.healthline.com/bug-bites)

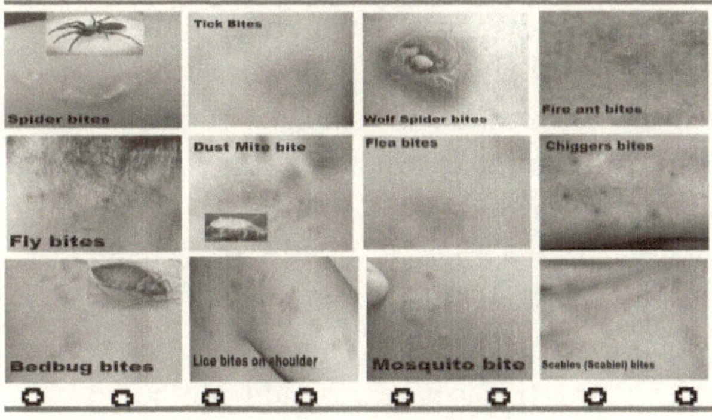

A real story, Tick bites killed a 3 years old child in 2016.

Where are those Tick BUGS come from?

Answer: They are outdoors for sure. Sometimes, they are inside of the house. See below pictures (Ref.: healthfacts.os.tc).

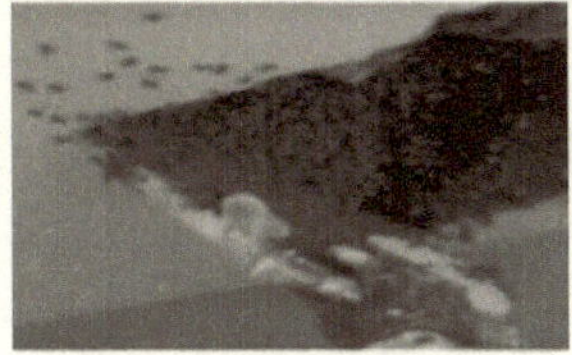

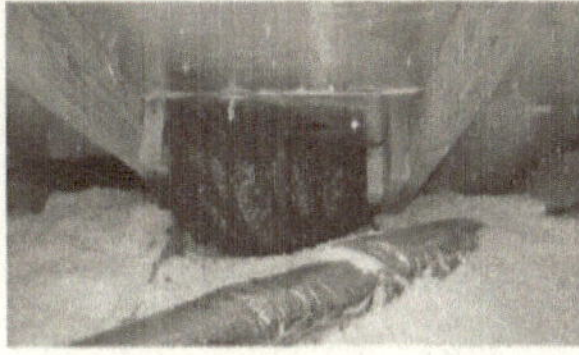

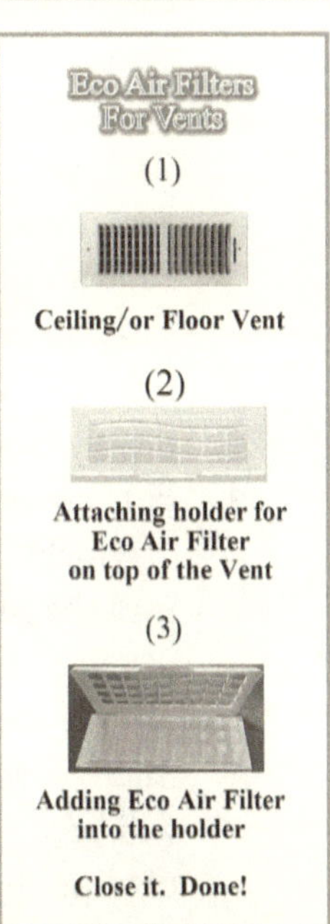

ECO-SAFE AIR FILTER MANUFACTURING CO.

Phone: 1 (678) 900-6617
Email: sales@EcosafeAirFilters.com
Site: www.EcosafeAirFilters.com

Removing the Odors at Home

Sometimes we smell something bad at home. We must find out what is making the bad smell and get things cleaned out to maintain good family health.

Here are a few tips for removing odors at home:

a) For removing odors in the refrigerator, put an opened box of baking soda in the refrigerator. This can also help keep food fresh for a longer time.

b) For removing the odor from shoes, put a few pieces of the old-fashioned mothballs into the *shoe* closet or shoeboxes. Sometimes, the odor is inside the shoes due to sports activities that people's feet sweat into the shoes. The wet condition could make the shoes smell bad. Treatment: Use a hammer to mash a few pieces of the moth balls and put some of the moth balls' powder inside each shoe. And put the shoes under the sunlight during noontime for two to three hours. It will remove the odor completely from your shoes.

c) For removing odors in the microwave oven, put a half cup of vinegar into a microwaveable bowl then put the bowl into the microwave oven. Then use it on *high* for one minute to heat the vinegar. If it is necessary, add another minute on the *high* setting. You will notice the odors in the microwave oven have disappear. Plus, the microwave oven will become amazingly easy to clean. Use a warm wet towel to wipe the inside of the microwave oven after.

Here are a few tips for removing odors on human body:

a) For removing odors in your hair, put two to three spoonfuls of baking soda into a large pot of warm water and stir it slowly until it dissolves into the water completely. Soak your hair into the mixture and gently rub the scalp and comb through the hairs for about ten minutes. Then use shampoo to wash your hair as you usually do. Repeat it every day for two to three days until the hair odor is removed.

b) For removing the odor in your mouth, brush your teeth in the morning and before bedtime. Use a hydrogen peroxide topical solution (a first aid antiseptic oral debriding agent) or use the refreshing mint mouthwash and gargle solution to gargle for two to three minutes right after brushing your teeth in the morning and before bedtime. It is important that do not eat any food or candy after cleaning your mouth at bedtime.

c) Option 1: chewing a few pieces of roasted peanuts in the daytime when you smell bad breath coming out.

Option 2: chewing a Doublemint bubble gum can help keep the bad smell away from the mouth.

d) When a person reaches puberty, special hormones affect the glands in the armpits. These glands make sweat that can really smell. Use armpit deodorant that has twenty-four-hour protection every day. And especially during the summertime, take a shower and roll a little deodorant onto your armpits as often as needed.

CHAPTER 2

Keep Your Body Clean and Healthy

Based on medical research and study, our hands might contain some bacteria and germs through working and touching something unclean. If we eat food with the uncleaned hands, the chances are taking some of the bacteria and germs into your stomach. It might cause stomach ache, running stomach, bugs in stomach, etc.

I highly advise you to do the following to stay away from getting sick often.

a) Use soap to wash your hands before eating meals.
b) Take a warm/hot shower with soap each day.
c) Drink a half cup of warm salt water (add a little bit of salt) after you get up in the morning. It helps clean your stomach.
d) Drink green tea in the morning during/after breakfast.

Treat an Itchy and/or Painful Throat

If you feel an itch inside your throat and you're sneezing, it happens when you breathe in some dusty air or allergy air through your nose and mouth; you need to take care yourself immediately. Use hydrogen peroxide (first aid antiseptic oral debriding agent) as an oral gargle and rinse agent. See the referenced product picture below.

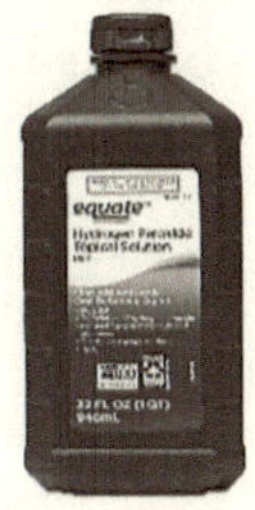 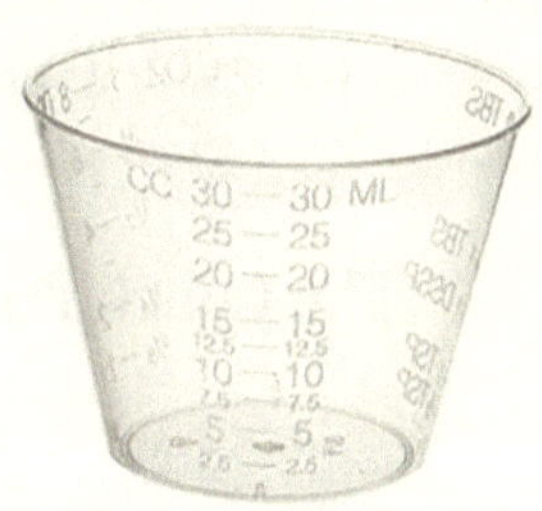

These are the directions for use: fill a cup with 15 mL of the solution, swish the undiluted solution in your mouth for one minute, then spit out the solution. Do this after breakfast and before bedtime while you have itchy and pain throat or bleeding gums while brushing your teeth. Or use it as needed when you feel the itch and pain.

Treat Itchy and Painful Nostrils

Use hydrogen peroxide (topical solution USP) as a *cleansing solution* when your *nostrils* feel itch and pain.

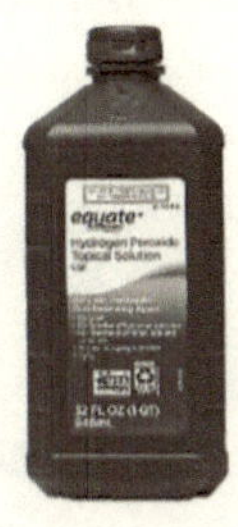 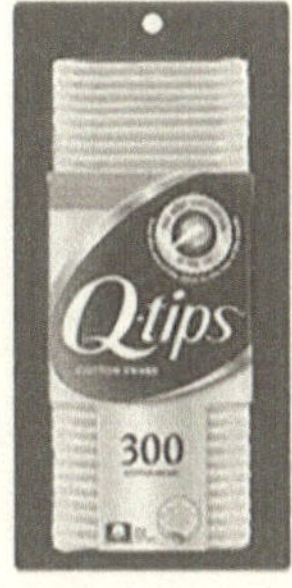

These are the directions for use: put a small amount of the hydrogen peroxide into a small container, dip two cotton swabs into the solution to wet the cotton, then use the soaked cotton swabs to clean each nostril. You will see white things being cleaned out, which is normal. Clean it often as needed to stop the itch and pain in your nostrils.

Hydrogen peroxide acts as a first aid antiseptic for the treatment of minor cuts and abrasions.

Most of the time, we felt our throat itchy and pain because of cold. For example, when the weather changes from summer to fall season, we haven't added more clothes yet the cold air blows on our body that makes us feel cold.

The Quick Recovery Method for Cold

1. Making some ginger tea to drink while it's hot/warm. Rest well in the bed for a few hours to recover yourself fast. You can stop the cold within one day when you treat it at the very beginning. Otherwise, it takes a week of time to recover from cold symptoms, such as running nose, cough, pain throat, headache, etc.

   Preparation: Cutting the ginger (2–5 g) to small pieces. Boil it in the pot with a full bowel of water. When the water is boiling, turn the stove to low heat to continue cook the ginger for ten minutes. Add a half spoonful of dark-brown sugar right after you take it off from the stove. The ginger tea is ready. Drink it when it's warm.
2. Putting some warm clothes on when you go outdoors.

Treat Skin That's Itchy from Bugbites

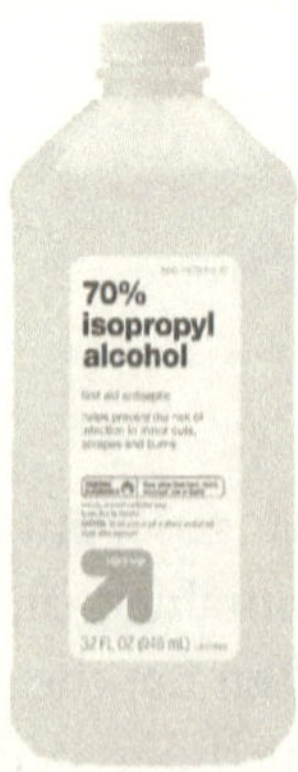

70 percent isopropyl alcohol

Use 50–70 percent isopropyl alcohol (also called rubbing alcohol) to rub your skin where you got bitten by a mosquito or some other tiny bug if you feel it's itchy. It will help to stop the itch.

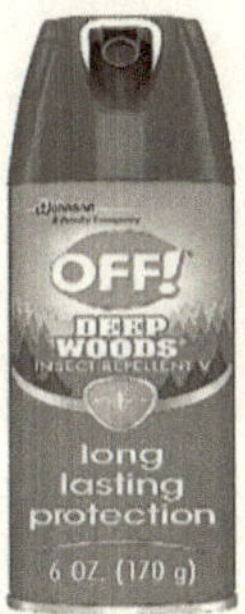

Deep Woods insect repellent

Use OFF! Deep Woods insect repellent to prevent bugbites. Spray some of the insect repellent on your body before going outdoors.

Mosquito bites usually leave a big bump on the bitten spot, and it can make you scratch yourself until you break your skin. For persistent itching on the skin due to bugbites, use hydrogen peroxide (topical solution USP) as a *cleansing solution* for the affected area. It can help stop the itching and act as an antiseptic.

The hydrogen peroxide topical solution is a particularly important first aid antiseptic oral debriding agent for people who live in the southern part of the United States such as South Carolina, Georgia, Alabama, Texas, Florida, etc. The hot and humid weather during the summer months create a rich environment for bugs and bacteria to grow.

In southern part of the United States, things in the *air* start appearing during the springtime. The wind blows pollen into the air, and this can land everywhere—on streets, on cars, on roofs, etc. It can cause allergies in people's eyes, noses, skin, etc.

We also see some tiny spiders and other kinds of tiny bugs that are sized like a little dot or a period in writing. When those little bugs have been blown onto people's skin/clothes when we go under trees or closer to an area with trees, they could cause people's skin to itch.

Those tiny spiders have colors like red, light yellow, semiclear white, and black. They can make people's skin itch and cause red dots to appear.

Therefore, we must keep up with the cleaning maintenance to keep a clean and healthy body.

Treat Sunburned Skin

Use sunscreen lotion to prevent sunburn. I suggest the Waterproof Sunscreen Lotion Intensive UV Sunblock cream— SPF50 + Moisturizing Skin. During the summer, we sweat a lot. The waterproof sunscreen lotion could help us stay away from sunburn for the whole day.

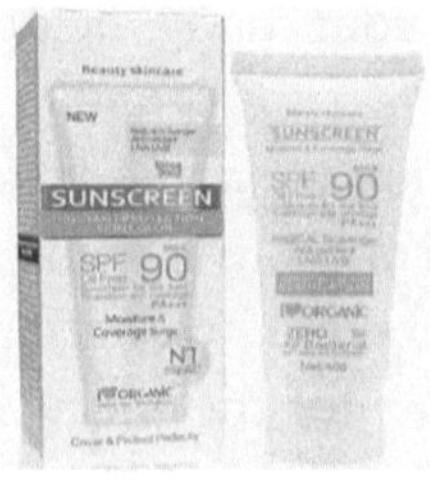

Waterproof sunscreen lotion

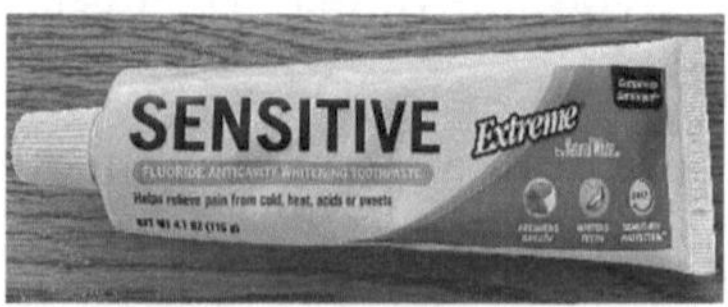

Toothpaste for sensitive teeth

This special *Sensitive* Extreme toothpaste from Natural White can help relieve pain from cold, heat, acids, or sweets in the gums (medically called "gingiva").

We can also use the toothpaste for a small patch of itchy or painful skin from minor burns due to sunburns, hot water, hot oil. It not only *stops pain* in the gums and pain in the skin due to minor cuts but can also *stop the itchy feeling* on the skin due to insect bites and sunburns.

Treat Itch or Pain at the Anus

The anus (also called asshole) is the opening in a person's bottom through which solid waste leaves the body. It might get irritated by the waste from time to time each day that causing it to itch or feel painful.

You can keep it clean and treat the itch/pain when it occurs by using Epsom salt. You will need the following items in the pictures show below:

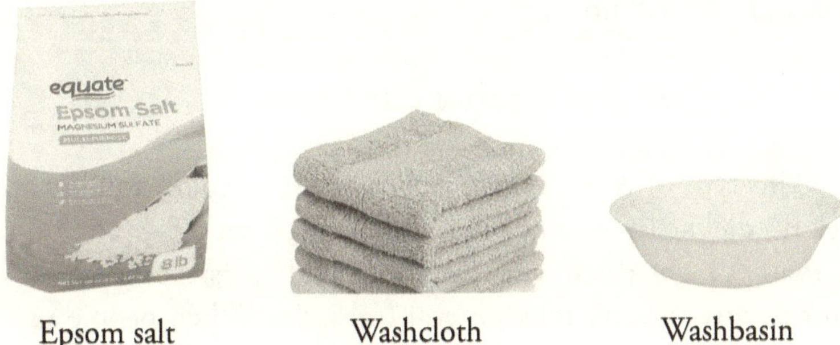

Epsom salt   Washcloth   Washbasin

Epsom salt (magnesium sulfate) is usually used when soaking minor sprains and bruises. Now we use Epsom salt to stop the anus itching.

a) Grab a handful of Epsom salt and put it in the washbasin (the size of washbasin should be large enough for you to soak your bottom in).

b) Get a small washcloth and fill the washbasin one-thirds full of hot water to dissolve the Epsom salt in.

c) When the temperature is warm enough to soak your hand in, soak your bottom in the warm/hot water for ten minutes in the washbasin.

d) Use the small washcloth to gently clean the itchy or painful place while it is soaked in the warm Epsom salt water.

For women, if your vulva is itchy, use a washcloth to clean the itchy spot while it is soaked in the warm/hot Epsom salt water until it stops feeling itchy.

Remember to check the temperature of the Epsom salt water. It should be around 70–75 °C (Celsius) or 158–167 °F (Fahrenheit). Based on research data, E. coli and most bacteria lose their activity when the temperature goes up to 75 °C.

The temperature of boiling water is 100 °C, which can burn your hand, so a temperature of 70–75 °C would not burn your hand or butt. You will feel the warmth when you test the water with your hand, but you will not get burned by it.

Treating Pinworms

This type of worm is very tiny, is white in color, and has a little black needlelike tip on one of its ends. It is about 0.5–1 cm long and less than 0.1 cm thick, and the other end is its reproductive side; it moves this around, making you feel itchy. When people use fingers to scratch it, the worm's eggs and/or larvae will be attach to the skin on your fingers. If people use their fingers to eat food, the eggs and/or larvae will go back into their stomachs and become the adult worm, and this can cause the anus to feel itchy again. That is the life cycle of the pinworm.

It is particularly important that people must wash their hands after using the bathroom to poop. Poop is also called excrement or shit.

Poop is an incredibly good source of nutrition for plants. It is commonly used to grow vegetables, flowers, and trees.

There are two treatment methods for pinworms. To stop the pinworm from causing the itchy anus, smooth a *big chunk of petroleum jelly on the anus* after washing and soaking with the warm Epsom salt-water solution. Petroleum jelly can stop the worm from moving around and therefore stop the itch.

Based on medical studies, these kinds of bug problems at the anus happened when we eat raw vegetables and when we eat food with fingers without washing our hands.

To avoid getting the worm from food, we can steam the vegetables or cook vegetables with meat for meals.

Always wash fruit with warm salt water then add a small spoonful of flour and soak in five minutes. Then wash and rinse with cold water.

Once you've stopped the worms from coming into your body through the mouth and fingers, one or two weeks later, you wouldn't have the anus itch problem that was caused by the pinworm.

Treat the itchy spot as often as needed.

CHAPTER 3

Keep Your Body's Immune System Strong

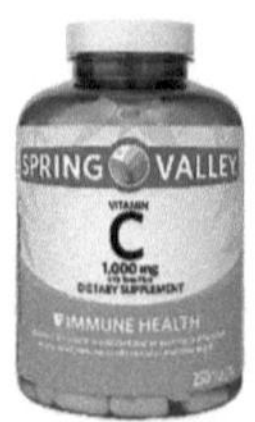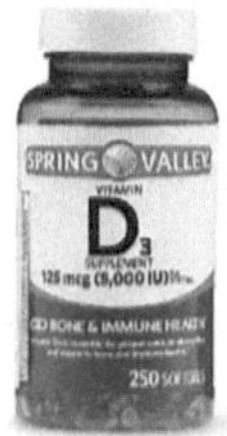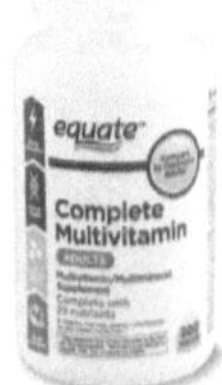

1. Take one piece of complete multivitamin per day.
2. Take one piece of vitamin C daily to boost the immune system.
3. Take one piece of vitamin D3 daily to increase the bone and immune health. I highly recommend you add a piece of vitamin C and a piece of vitamin D3 in addition to your regular complete multivitamin supplement to boost your immune system so that the coronavirus has a lesser chance of making you sick.
4. Chicken soup: make chicken soup at home once per week for your body and soul.
5. Eat more *beans*. Most beans contain some isoflavones, which have a combination of wrinkle-reducing isoflavones. It helps your body stay young.

6. Eat three meals per day regularly. Eat more at lunchtime and less during dinnertime.
7. Reenergize your body by taking thirty to sixty minutes to rest/nap after lunch.

CHAPTER 4

Onion Treatment to Stop Fainting/Dizziness

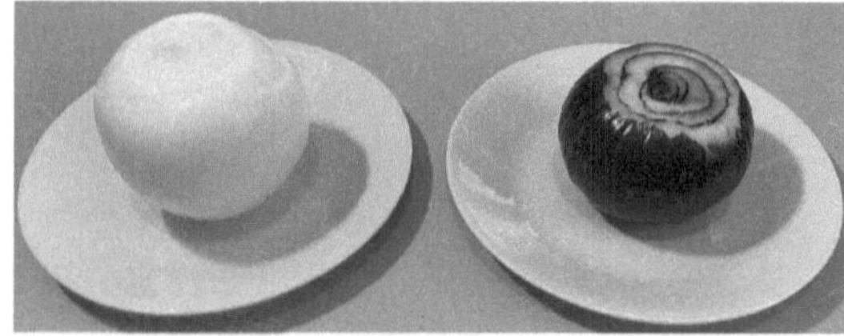

Yellow or purple

It doesn't matter as long as they are onions.

When you feel a little bit of shortness of breath, dizzy, and a slight cough (any one of the symptoms), do the onion treatment.

Cut a fresh onion (see pictures). Smell and breathe in the onion's odor from nose; take a deep breath down to the chest then breathe it out from mouth. Do it twenty times. It can stop people from fainting.

Based on the herb study, the onion's odor can keep away germs that might possibly be attached to the walls/membranes inside our respiratory system. Some areas include inside the nostrils, the throat, the lungs, etc.

After smelling it, put the onion by your bedside. The onion can absorb some germs in the air and keep them away from you.

CHAPTER 5

Food Medicines

Food medicines are useful in maintaining good health and treating symptoms at the beginning for fast healing and recovery. If you have a seriousness/severe combination of medical issues, I advise you to see a doctor.

3 Methods That Can Stop Coughing

Coughing is the most common symptom that people experience when they feel sick. Here I share the three most efficient food medicines for treating cough.

Method 1: rock sugar and pear juice

Materials include one pear and a few pieces of rock sugar.

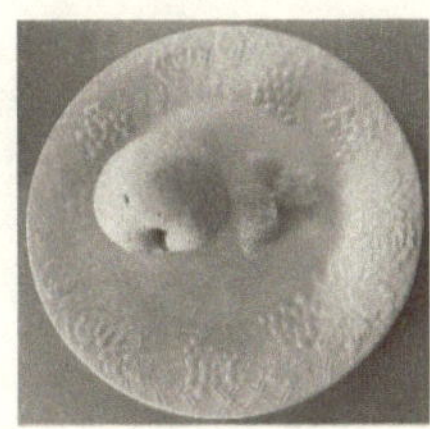

One pear and pieces
of rock sugar

→

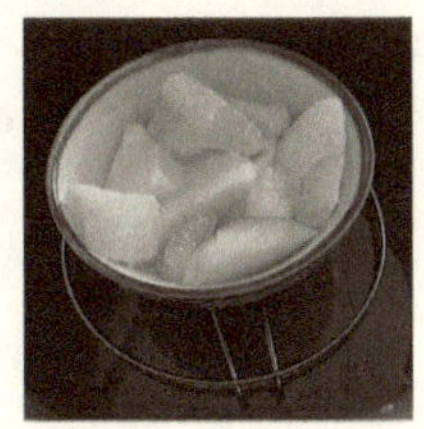

Prepare to steam in pot

Cut the pear to smaller pieces and take the core out. Steam the pear and a few pieces of rock sugar with a bowl full of water together (see pictures above) for fifteen minutes. Eat the pear and drink the juice when it is warm. Eat this for a continued three to five days as light refreshment and rest well. You will feel your lungs getting clearer and better each day when you do deep breaths. You should be healed from the cough.

Method 2: garlic juice

Materials include: seven cloves of garlic and a few pieces of rock sugar.

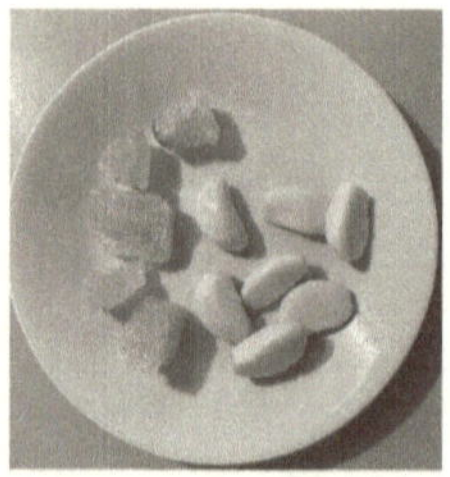

Seven pieces of garlic
and some rock sugar

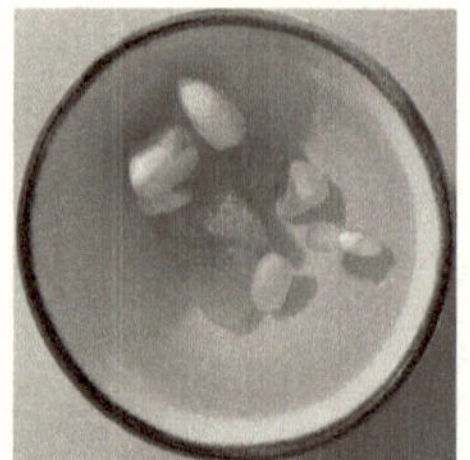

Prepare to steam for
fifteen minutes

You can also cut or grinding the garlic into small pieces if you don't like to bite on the whole garlic piece. The juice in the garlic is also the key element for food medicine. Make sure you save the garlic juice for your garlic tea. Steam the garlic and a few pieces of rock sugar with a bowl full of water together (see pictures above) for fifteen minutes. You will see the rock sugar melt out into the garlic juice. Drink the juice when it is warm.

Method 3: eggplant's base juice

Materials include a few eggplants' base parts.

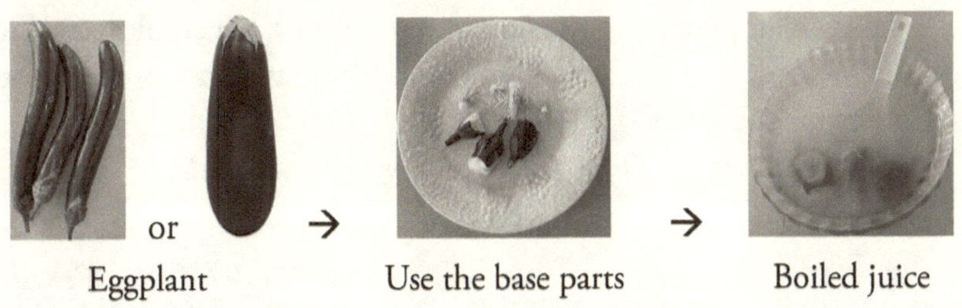

Eggplant   Use the base parts   Boiled juice

Boil the eggplants' base parts (roots from green onion are optional) in a full bowl of water (about 0.75 L) in a pot for fifteen minutes. Drink the juice when it is warm. Do this in the morning. You can drink it twice per day; just boil it again in the afternoon. Use fresh base parts for next day. Take this continuously for three to five days and rest well. The cough will stop. Some people said it stopped their many years of chronic cough. Eggplant is an edible vegetable and is safe for everybody in the family to try, including young children.

Clean Your Body's Blood Clots

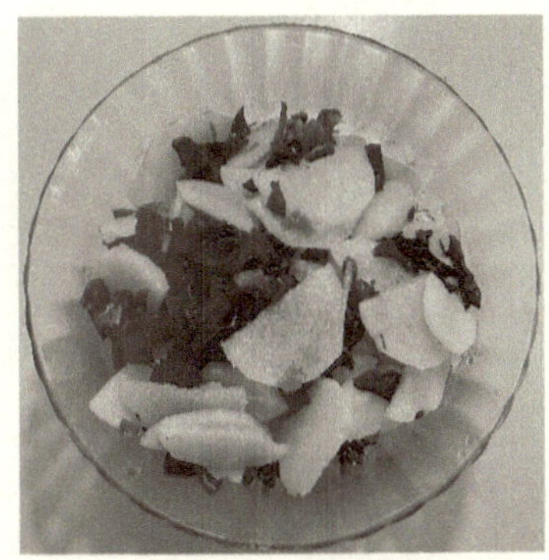

Wood ear cooked with common yam

Materials include wood ear fungus. The wood ear fungus is an herbal medicine ingredient that has been recorded hundreds of years ago in Chinese herbal medicine books.

Here we emphasize on the benefit of wood ear; they can reduce and clean blood clots from the human body. You can add the wood ear to meat soup, cook it with egg, or cook with vegetables. Eating wood ear keeps your body strong and healthy, which can help you stay safe from the COVID-19 pandemic.

Here are instructions for preparing the raw materials:

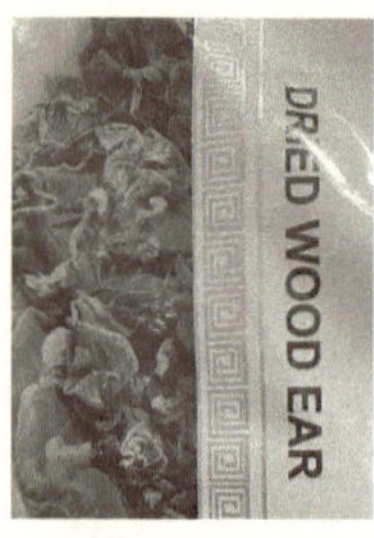

Dried wood ear

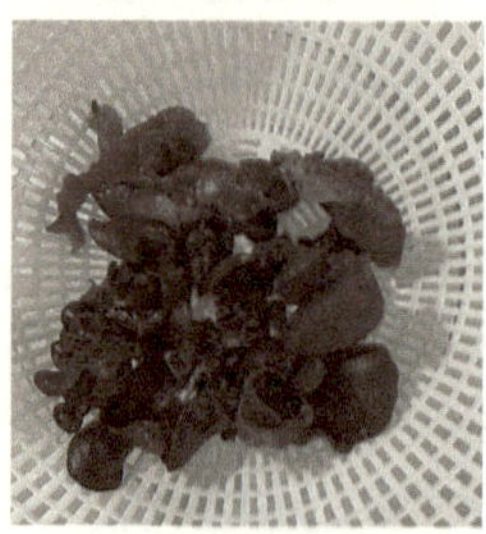

Soak in water
for two hours

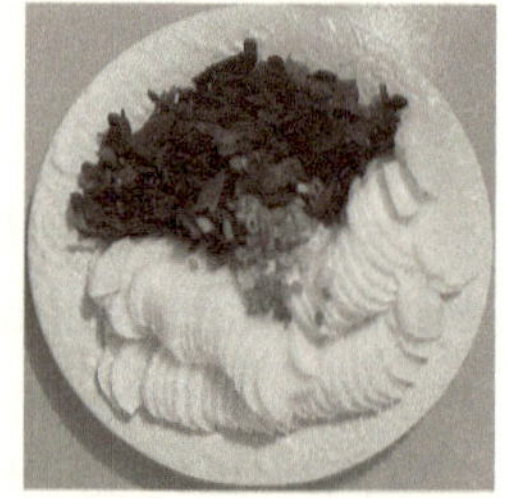

Cut it into smaller
pieces for cooking

Grab a handful of wood ear (about 1 gram) and soak it in a bowl of warm water. After one to two hours, you will see it enlarge and become soft, like in the picture shown above.

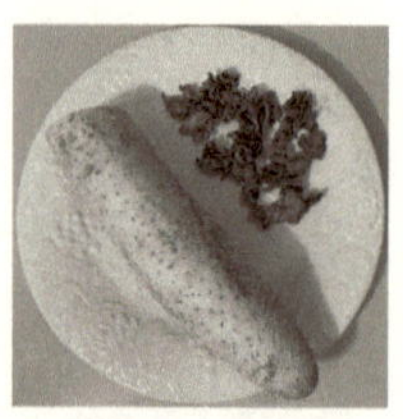

Dried wood ear
Common yam
(rhizome)

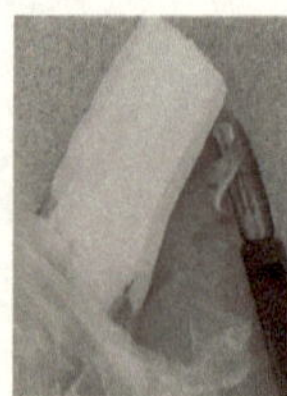

Peel the skin

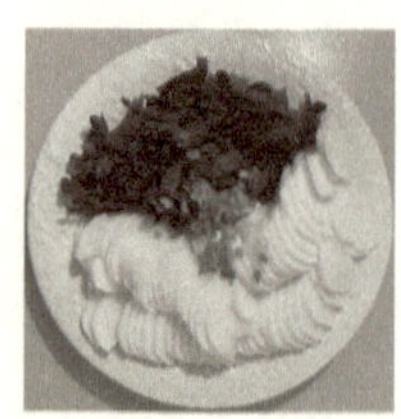

Slices for cooking

When you peel the skin from the yam, hold it with a plastic bag. There are some pointy things on the yam's skin that may make your hand feel itchy.

The common yam (rhizome) has the core function of promoting digestion and blood circulation. It also can lower blood sugar, benefit the lungs, and relieve cough. Additionally, it can aid in the prevention of cardiovascular and cerebrovascular diseases; yam is rich in mucus protein, vitamins, and trace elements, which can well inhibit the deposition of blood lipids onto the vascular wall, playing the role of being pro-longevity.

Foods That Make the Immune System Strong

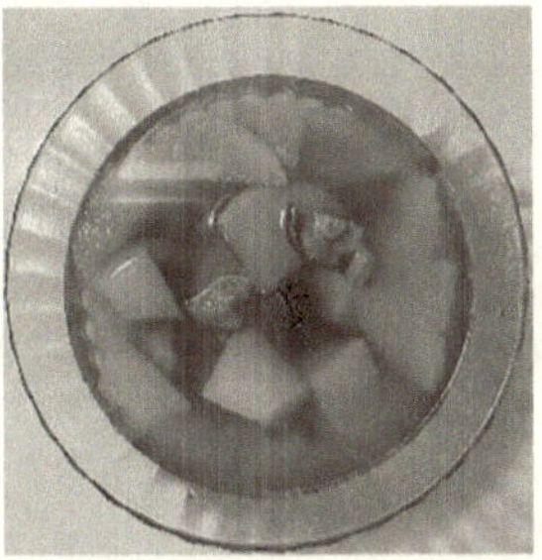

White radish and mushroom soup

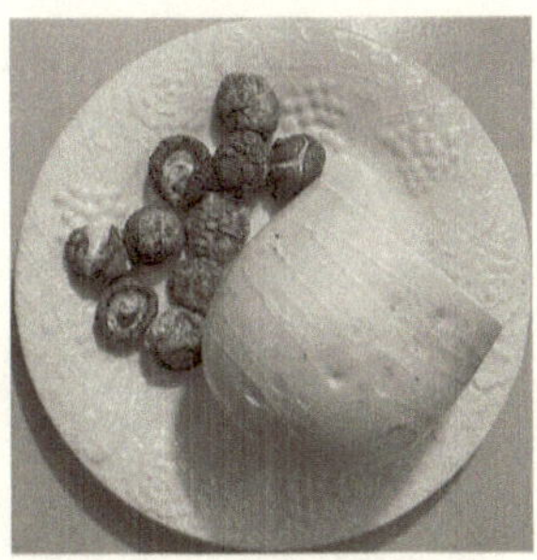

Here are instructions on how to prepare the white radish and dried mushrooms: Soak the dried mushrooms in warm water for two to three hours in a bowl. You can check it if it is ready for cook or not by cutting it in the middle. When it becomes soft inside the root part, it is ready for cooking. Cut the white radish into smaller pieces that you like for your soup.

The following are benefits of consuming white radish:

a) *Prevention of cancer.* The cellulose in white radish helps the body discharge metabolic waste and maintain a healthy state. In addition, the lignin in white radish can decompose ammonium nitrite in the blood. Ammonium nitrite is the harmful substance that causes cell cancelation. Edible white radish can help anybody eliminate cancer cells, thus having the effect of cancer prevention.

b) *Cools the blood to prevent bleeding.* White radish is cooling. It can get rid of lung heat and treat oral ulcers caused by heat toxin in the body, sores in the mouth and tongue, a dry pharynx by having it sweat, and other symptoms. Many people get headache or feeling a heavy head because of overdrinking alcoholic products. White radish can help reduce the problem.

c) *Promotes digestion.* The cellulose content in white radish is rich; it can promote gastrointestinal peristalsis, help the digestive tract discharge metabolic waste, and increase appetite to help digestion. It can also help purge and acts as a diuretic. It can treat inappetence. Additionally, it can stop cough and dissolve phlegm.

Caution: Do not eat white radish and wood ear in the same meal. It might cause skin allergies. Do not eat it with apples in the same meal.

The following are benefits of consuming mushrooms:

a) Mushrooms can efficiently reduce blood pressure, delay senility, and prevent constipation.

b) Mushrooms are antiaging. The new technology proves that the juice extracted from mushroom can make skin beautiful and antiaging.

c) Mushrooms also play a therapeutic role in diabetes, tuber-
culosis, infectious hepatitis, and neuritis and can be used
for indigestion, constipation, and other diseases.

Caution: Do not cook and eat it with tomatoes and/or carrots
in the same meal. It may reduce the nutrition on both foods, and you
can lose the benefits of mushroom.

CHAPTER 6

Aromatherapy and Massage Therapy

When you are very tired and/or have body pain due to heavy body-work or working long hours, your immune system becomes weak. You must get good rest to recover yourself.

I suggest you try aromatherapy and combine it with massage therapy; use this on the painful parts of your body. Do it with your family members or friends, depending on your situation.

The research shows that people can quickly recover and recharge by massaging with a pleasant, fragrant smell and/or soothing aromatherapy scents like in body oil. You may also listen to soft sounds of calming background music or ocean sounds while you rest for the night. A well-rested sleep could reenergize your body to work more efficiently for the new day. The best amount of sleep is at least eight hours at night. Try to sleep before 10:00 p.m., and you should wake up at 6:00 a.m. Based on medical research, data have shown that human body are self-repairing the organs while you are asleep during 11:00 p.m. to 3:00 a.m.

With one exception, for example, when we travel to other countries that have six- to ten-hour-time differences, we might find ourselves still in the sleeping schedule that we get used to. It will take three days to a week of time to adjust the physiological time difference. It means that our body has the ability to adjust itself. Some people work at night shift schedules; they developed their new routine sleeping cycles.

However, keeping a regular schedule of work and rest is important and guarantees good health.

Taking a thirty-minute to a one-hour nap after lunch is also a particularly important way to reenergize your body for the afternoon.

Self-Massages on Hands for Healing

Massaging your hands daily may provide a good maintenance for your five viscera and six entrails, based on traditional Chinese medicine and studies on acupuncture points.

The Chinese public health education (see the referenced pictures below) teaches us that there are many acupuncture points on the hands that are connected to internal organs of the body such as the heart, spleen, liver, lungs, and kidneys.

When we feel some symptoms in the body, we can massage both hands entirely and focus on the specific area that reflects the corresponding body part to prevent a serious sickness from happening.

rectum
anus
ovary
kidney
bladder
ovary
kidney
spleen
large intestine
cecum
small intestine
liver
pancreatic
lung
heart
stomach
trachea
bronchial
esophagus

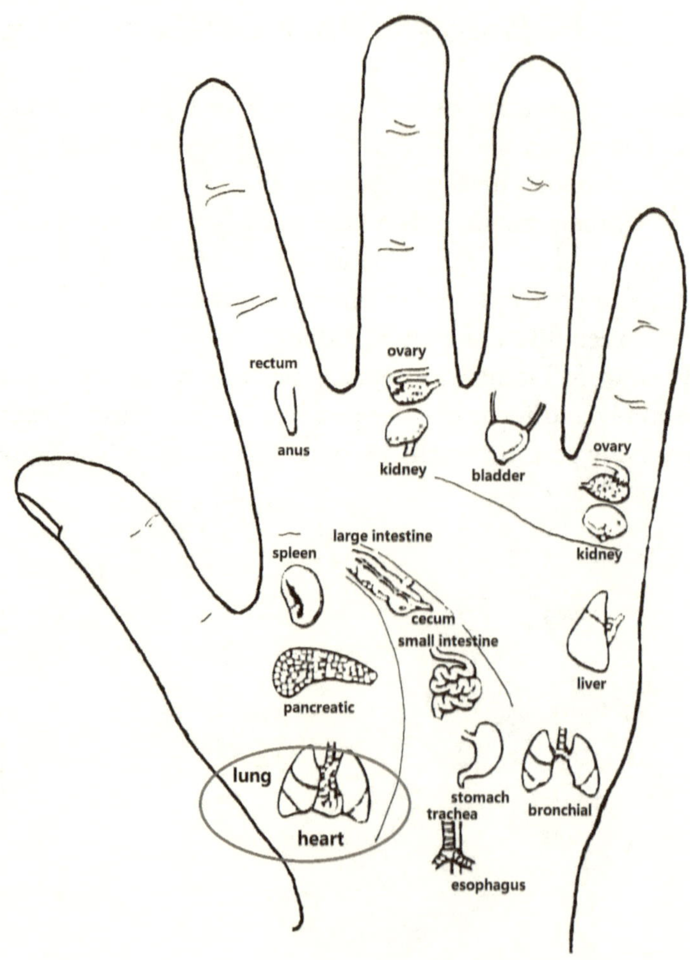

Left Hand

wrist
elbow
wrist
elbow
ankle
knee
ankle
knee
coxa
brain
hypophysis
coxa
shoulder
eye, ear, nose
Massage here
daily 10 min.
mouth, throat,
thyroid gland
esophageal
spleen
breathe system
stomach
liver
neck
pancreatic
chest
small
intestine
duodenum
colon
waist
urinate
kidney
shit
kidney
rectum
caudal vertebrae
anus
cardiovascular
system
genitals

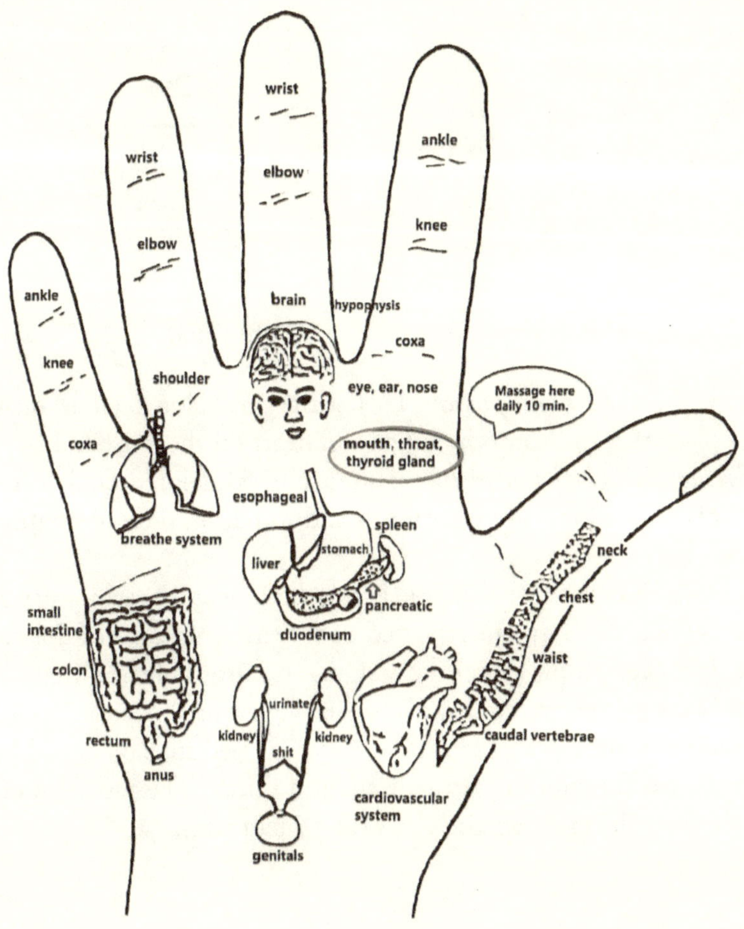

Right Hand

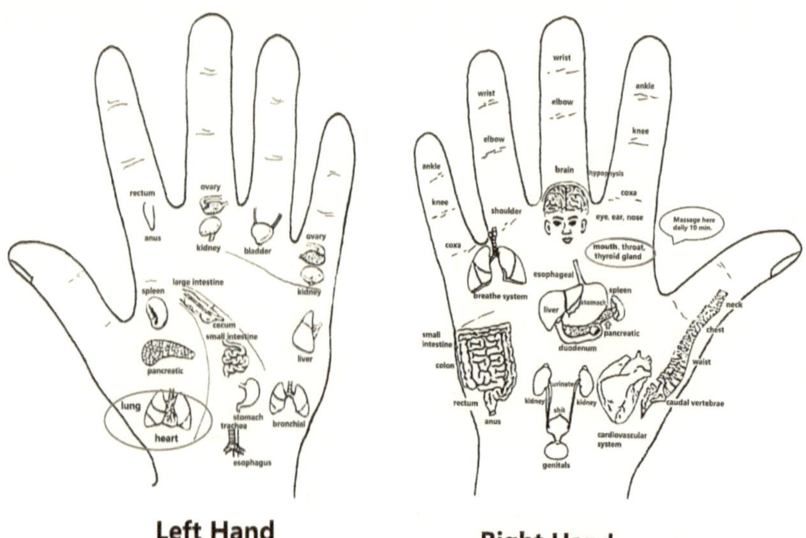

Left Hand   **Right Hand**

Reference 1: Left hand picture: I used the red-colored circle on the place that indicates the lungs and heart on the left hand.

Reference 2: Right hand picture: I used the red-colored circle on the place that indicates the mouth and throat on the right hand.

The COVID-19 pandemic is attacking people's respiratory system, as what the hospitals reported about the symptoms of this sickness. It makes people sick; they cough and cannot breathe well.

Massage the two circled places on the hands above for ten minutes in the morning and ten minutes before bedtime. This will help improve the functioning of the lungs and throat. Therefore, you can stay healthy during/after the COVID-19 pandemic.

CHAPTER 7

Daily Exercise

There are many types of exercises that people do to stay healthy. The most common exercises are yoga, Tai chi, and health exercises. Yoga is a good discipline for learning to relax. Yoga is usually combined with meditation to stay mentally calm. Tai chi is an ancient form of self-defenses. It focuses on internal Qi to circulate inside the body.

At school, from elementary to high school, we do health exercises and eye exercises at 10:00 a.m. which is between the four classes in the morning.

No matter what kind of exercise that you do, do one daily to stay healthy.

Some people like to do their yoga before sleeping at night. Occasionally, I do exercise at night before sleeping. If I missed my morning exercise due to busy schedule, I always make it up with some house work like sweeping the floor, mopping the floor, cleaning the kitchen, etc.

There are three basics daily physically exercises for staying healthier:

1. Get up in the morning and do the body stretching exercise that you usually do.
2. Walk at least thirty minutes per day.
3. There are many acupuncture points on our two hands that can treat shoulder pain, neck pain, and other types of body

pain. Doing some self-massage on your hands' acupuncture points will help you stay healthy.

Exercise is good for the brain. Exercise can be done in two forms: (1) exercising your body through work such as yard work, sweeping the floor, mopping the floor, etc. and (2) exercising at a fitness center.

When your body has movement, it makes your heart actively pump blood through your blood vessels. It keeps your body active and healthy.

This exercise strategy is especially important for people who work in the office and/or at home. Doing some exercise each day can help you stay healthy and get work done more efficiently.

CHAPTER 8

Treat Dark Spots and Skin Tags

Some of the most common skin issues are dark spots, skin tags, freckles, age spots, moles, warts, etc. As a matter of fact, everyone wants to have clean and beautiful skin, especially on the face. The good news is technology is developing, and many new and improved products are available in the market to help people resolve those skin issues.

Freckles are caused by long-term exposure from sunlight for teenagers. For older adults, we see some age spots on the hands, arms, and face. I have tested many products. I suggest using *PFMC Fade Cream* to treat freckles and age spots. If the brown spot cannot be removed by the cream, try the *skin tag remover*. The skin tag remover can help remove moles and warts as well. See product pictures below for your reference.

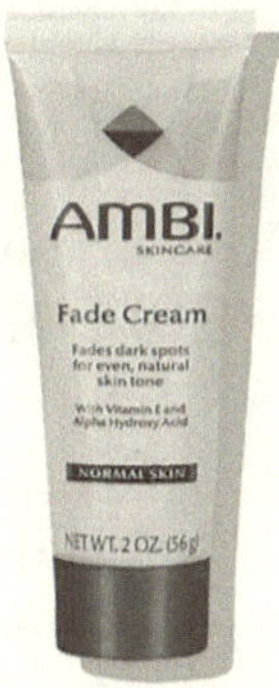

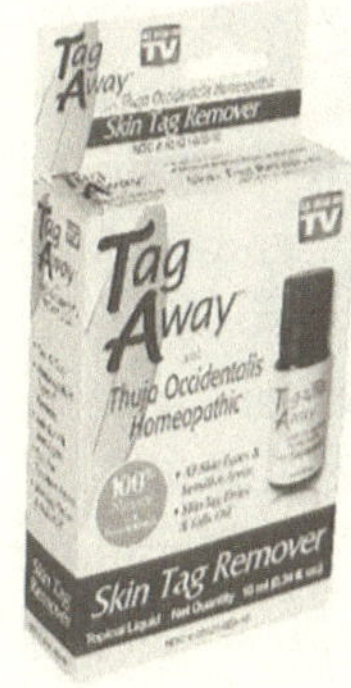

Pimples are caused by the hair follicle being blocked by the oil on the skin's surface. Acne is caused by clogged follicles. It shows some oil and dead skin cells leading to whiteheads and blackheads. Acne and pimples come and go as we keep up the treatment on the face. It associated with meals, especially when you eat a big meal with fried chicken or any food that has a lot of fatty parts on it.

These are some solutions:

a)   Eat less fatty meat and more vegetables; this will improve the acne skin.
b)   Drinking green tea will help remove some extra fat from the meals that we have eaten.
c)   Use the skins of fruit (the inside part) to massage the face to remove the extra oil that accumulated during the day from exploring to outdoor activities. Use fruits such as banana, orange, apple, and watermelon.

Use banana skin to treat warts on the face. Use the inside part of banana skins to massage the face, especially the wart. Slowly you might see an improvement and get clearer skin on your face.

Use homemade skin-fading solution to remove the dark-colored spots. You will need the following materials:

a)   one egg (use the white part only and take the yolk out)
b)   one inch of toothpaste (whitening formula)
c)   two spoonfuls of vinegar
d)   two spoonfuls of milk

Mix them well.

Before you take a shower before going to bed, rub the homemade fading solution (liquid) on your face, neck, and arms and gently massage your skin for about ten to twenty minutes, then wash it out with warm water.

Put a small amount of lotion on your skin before sleeping.

You will see a significant result of clearer and lighter skin on your face after you continuously use it for one month.

CHAPTER 9

Healing Dry Skin and Skin Maintenance

Dry skin can be healed by putting petroleum jelly on the skin every day after washing and/or showering.

If the skin on your whole body is feeling dry and itchy and if you see some white skin flaking or creasing due to dryness, you can use moisturizing soap to wash your body. Then apply some baby oil or coconut body oil on your skin and massage it for about ten minutes without rinsing it out.

Continue the petroleum jelly and body oil treatment for ten days. You will see a significantly improved result on your skin.

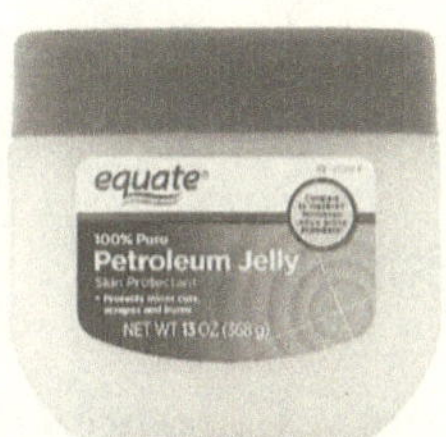

Petroleum jelly

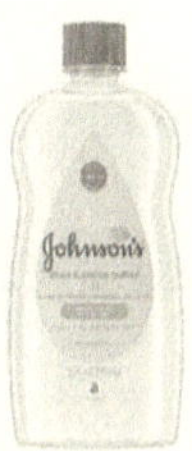

Baby oil

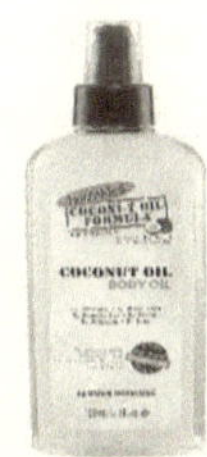

Coconut oil for the body

Homemade Moisturizing Water for Stopping Itch and Dry Skin

You will need the following materials:

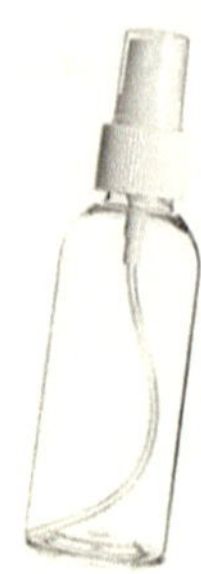

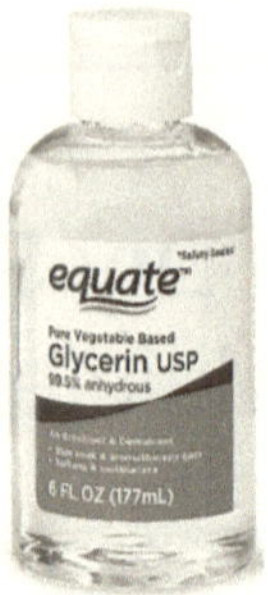

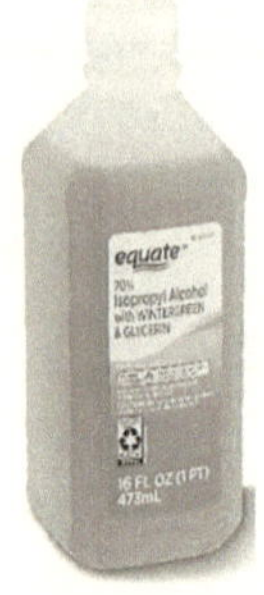

Spray bottle   Glycerin   Isopropyl alcohol

1. Grab an empty spray bottle.
2. Add purified drinking water into the bottle (80 percent of the bottle).
3. Add glycerin into the spray bottle (remaining 20 percent of the bottle).
4. Add 15 mL of 70 percent alcohol with wintergreen.
5. Mix them well, and it will be ready to use.

When you feel an itch on your skin, especially during the wintertime, you can spray some of your own homemade body moisturizing water on your skin to heal the dry skin and stop the itch.

Overall Skin Maintenance Methods

Treat mosquito bites during the summertime. Currently the most powerful product in the market for healing the mosquito bites is the Cutter Insect Repellent. I suggest you have at least two bottles handy for your family's needs during the summer each year.

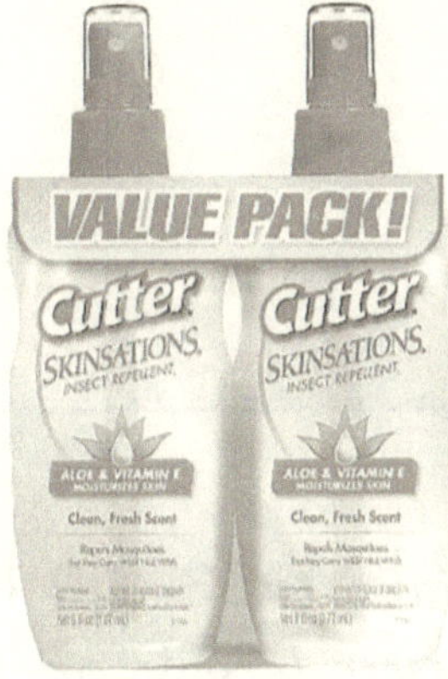

When you have skin rashes due to allergies or poisonous plants and are scratching on your legs or hands, use the over-the-counter medicine Cortizone-10.

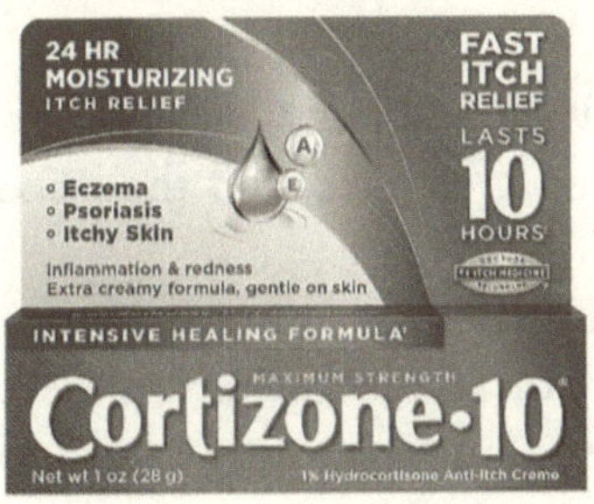

To avoid sunburn, put some sunblock lotion on the face, neck, arms, and legs where your skin is exposed to the sunlight. During the summertime, we often experience a sunburn situation when we go to beach to swim or hike in the mountains for outdoor activities.

CHAPTER 10

Facial Massage for a Younger-Looking Face

Getting a facial massage is a great method to keep skin tight and look young and beautiful for a longer time. *Use facial oil to massage your face.*

For reference, I selected a few facial oil products based on the function that we need it to have, and the prices are below $15 per bottle.

Caution: Avoid getting the oil into your eyes. In case you have a little oil in your eye by accident, rinse your eye with plenty of cold water for about five minutes. Putting a drop of the Opcon-A Eye Allergy Relief eye drops into each eye can help avoid eye irritation along with redness, itch, and allergy symptoms.

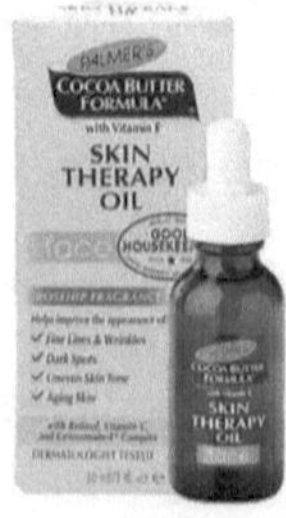

Palmer's Skin
Therapy Oil

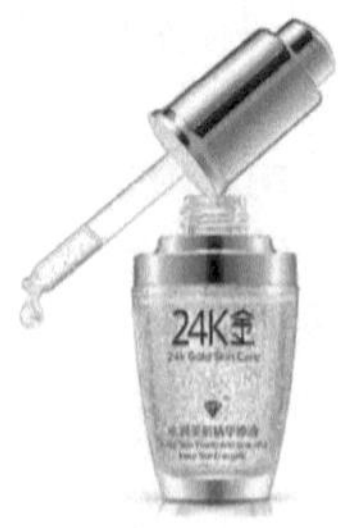

Antiaging face oil

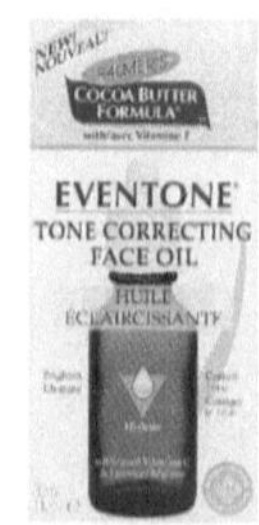

Tone-correcting
face oil

Here are different methods you can use for your facial massage:

1. To reduce eye bags, use the third finger (also called the ring finger) to put a drop of face oil on each eye bag and massage it, going from the eye's inner corner to the outer corner. Then move your fingers up a little to your eyelid and gently massage your eyelid skin from the outer corner to inner corner of the eye. Massage your eye by gently moving your third fingers around your eye. Softly move your finger around the eye for about ten times.

2. Massage the forehead with both hands from the center of forehead to each side. Do it ten times.

3. Use your two thumbs to massage the area behand each ear. Put a little bit of pressure on it and move up and down ten to twenty times.

4. Massage your cheeks with both hands. Starting from the jaw and chin, move slowly up to the top of your head. Do it ten times.

5. Use your index and middle fingers together to massage the point beside the nose. Move your two fingers at the same point in circle for ten times. Put a little pressure on the points to prevent rhinitis coryza (also called nasitis).

6. For students, use your index finger and the thumb to hold the glabella and eye socket and massage it. It can help you relax your eyes after a long hour of reading.

7. For girls, please avoid reading on the computer for long time when you have your monthly menstruation because the loss of blood might weaken your eyesight if you continuously use your eyes for more than two hours. Take a break and relax your eyes for ten minutes before going back to your desk to read again if you have to get some reading and writing work done.

8. Message your ears for a few minutes each day. Press your ears with your hands then release. You will feel the air being pumped out from the ears. It can help loosen some earwax.

9. Use both your middle fingers to massage the sides of your nose. From the sides of your nostrils, move up to the top of the forehead then move down to the sides of the nostrils again. Move slowly with a little pressure from the middle fingers. Do this ten times.

10. Use your ten fingers to comb your hair thoroughly from the forehead to the back end at neck. Do it ten times.

11. Massage your jaw, starting from the behind the ears to the jaw and chin. Use your right hand to massage the left side from behind the ear to the chin. Use your left hand to massage the right side from behind the ear part to the chin part.

CHAPTER 11

Eczema Treatment

Why do people have eczema? Eczema is mainly caused by genetic factors and environmental factors. Genetic factors are from inside the body; there is a protein has a genetic mutation. It can be passed down from parents to children. The external factors that trigger eczema include moist/humid/damp environments; this can damage the skin.

a) If the eczema is caused by living in a humid environment, you need to improve your living environment. For example, some people live in the basement rooms. It might cause them to have eczema, especially when their parent has a history of eczema. Genetically, they can get the eczema problem really fast when exposed to the moist/humid/damp environment.

b) If the eczema is caused by a lack of exercise and physical work/activity, you need to do some more exercise to help your body sweat out the extra water under your skin. Do remember to drink some water slowly during the physical work and sweat times to avoid dehydration.

c) If the eczema is caused by your sleeping schedule (for example, sleeping too late and not getting up in the morning on time), you need to change your daily schedule to have a healthy sleeping habit.

d) Do not overeat. Overeating will cause the problem of sub-cutaneous fat accumulation. When there is too much fat under the skin, it could block your sweat from coming out, which can cause metabolic disorders.

Here are some treatment methods for eczema:

a) Drink green tea in the morning after breakfast. Tea could help people's urinary system by urinating the excess water out.

   Note: Do not drink tea after 4:00 pm because the tea contains some theophylline which can make people awake for a few hours. Most people have the sleeping schedule at 9:00 p.m. or 10:00 p.m. We want to sleep well after the whole day's work and/or study without anything that might disturb our sleep.

b) Life needs water. We should have eight cups of water each day to maintain a good, healthy body. And the body will urinate the extra body waste out.

c) Eat three meals per day and on time with your daily schedule. Do not wait until you are hungry to eat. Eat meals at the standard hours. For example, breakfast is from 6:00 a.m. to 7:00 a.m. Lunch hour is from noon to 1:00 p.m. Dinnertime is during 6:00 p.m. to 8:00 p.m.

d) Use food medicine. Some vegetables and fruit are particularly good for digestion and can help the urinary system remove excess moisture, for example, radish, red beans, mung beans, peanuts, potatoes, carrots, ginger, millet, yellow corn, lotus seeds, pumpkin, yam, and so on.

e) Some fruits are good for the functioning of the spleen by removing the extra moisture in body, for example, watermelon, orange, mango, papaya, pineapple, yellow peach, sweet pear, banana, etc.

f) In addition, often stimulating and patting some associated acupuncture points that also can remove moisture.

CHAPTER 12

Hair Loss Treatment

The hair loss is caused by heredity, hormonal changes, or medical conditions and is also a normal part of aging. Excessive hair loss from your scalp can make you bald.

The most common reason is age. Have the confidence to have a beautiful hair again. There are many products available in the market now for growing your hair back.

I introduce to you the most economic and affordable (less than $8 per bottle) product: *Regrow 7-Day Ginger Germinal Hair Growth Serum Hair Loss Treatment Oil (30mL)*. See picture below.

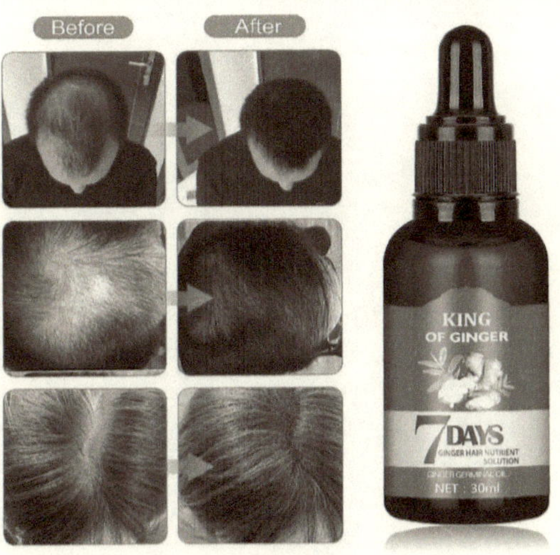

There are a few methods to maintain beautiful hair. There is also a method that we can use in our personal cleanliness to avoid the hair loss.

For oily hair, add a spoonful of baking soda to warm water and wash your hair with it once per week to remove the extra oil buildup from the scalp.

For dry hair, massage some olive oil or coconut oil into the ends of your hair, where the split ends are.

CHAPTER 13

Red Eye and Itchy Eye Treatment

Pink eye is a common disease that it is a type of bacterial infection. The symptoms are red and swollen eyes, itchy, painful, and/or dry eyes, pricking eye, excess tears, fear of light, more discharge than usual, etc. Giving timely treatment will help you recover soon.

It could be caused by pollen, dust, or something floating in the work environment that lands in your eyes. People always feel like wanting to rub with their hands when something irritates the eyes. Rubbing with unclean hands might make the eyelids swell and cause eye inflammation.

Here are some quick methods to resolve the situations:

a) Water rinse treatment: Rinse your eyes with clean water for a few seconds. Pat dry with a clean towel or paper towel with the eyes closed to avoid anything touching the eyes directly.

b) Use moisturizing eye drops or a redness-relief eye drop solution to clear the eyes. They are available at Walmart stores for $0.97 per 0.5 fl. oz. bottle. Put a few drops of moisturizing eye drops to clean out any particles out from the eyes. This works if you use it immediately after feeling the irritation.

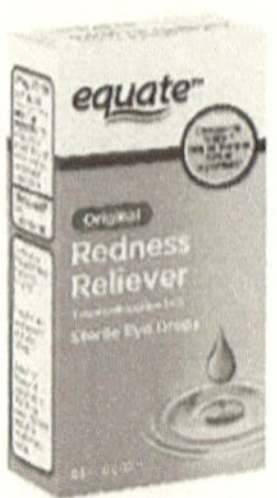

c) Use *eye allergy relief solution* to treat pink eye. When you have a large amount of sticky yellowish or white substance at the cornea, it can lead to blurred vision. Clean it out with a clean towel and warm water. Use the eye allergy relief eye drops immediately.

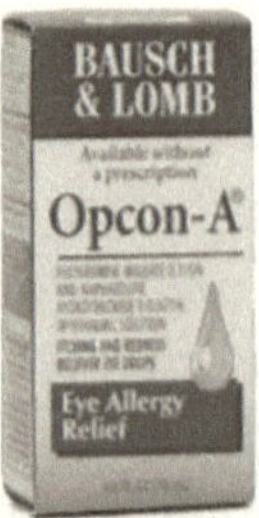

This is the most efficient eye allergy relief solution
that is available without a prescription.

Have good, healthy reading habits. Sit at a desk and keep at least one foot between your eyes and your reading target (such as computer screens and books).

CHAPTER 14

Hearing Health Maintenance

Deafness can be inherited, or it can be acquired due to inflammation or nerve disease. If you experience significant hearing loss, you must go to see doctors in the hospital for treatment to avoid serious damage to your hearing and permanent hearing impairment.

How do we maintain good hearing health?

a) Protect your ears daily. Avoid infection caused by dirty water entering the ears when you wash face and hair by using a clean cotton swab. Gently wipe the ear if you feel some water got into it.

b) Do not stay in a noisy environment often. Hearing loss could be caused by loud music and loud noises. If you work in construction industry or manufacturing industry, some machines make loud noises' you must use *earplug* that can help reduce the sound volumes of noise to protect your ears.

c) Some people like to use headset. You make sure the volumes is not too loud for your ears. You need to take breaks from the headset every two to three hours.

d) To remove earwax, use a cotton swab and wet the tip into a hydrogen peroxide topical solution (first aid antiseptic). Gently clean the earwax out. Usually, the earwax comes out itself without cleaning. You only need to clean it when you feel a little itch or irritation inside the ear.

e)   Massage your ears daily for five minutes. If you do health exercise daily, it should be included in the exercise already.

Step 1: Use your hands to rub both of ears up and down for ten times.

Step 2: Use your index fingers to gently insert to both ears and move around up and down two times and quickly take fingers out as you are taking a small piece of dried earwax out.

Step 3: Repeat step 2 twice.

CHAPTER 15

Car Sickness Treatment

Modern Medicine Method

Take a motion sickness pill before traveling by car or by airplane. For people who are wary of the side effects of medicine, the herb method might be the best option for car sickness treatment.

Herb Method

Put a slice of ginger on your belly button by taping it with a bandage. When you feel carsick, use your hand to push down on your belly button where the ginger is sitting then take deep breaths slowly; breathe in through your nose and breathe out through your mouth until the symptoms disappear.

Hand Massage Method

Use your thumb and index finger to hold the point (also called *hegu* point in traditional Chinese medical practice) between the opposite thumb and index finger. Use your right hand to massage your left hand. Then use your left hand to massage your right hand. Do it whenever you need it to stop feeling like throwing up from car sickness.

Fresh Air Method

Sit at the front seat and near the window if you have car sickness situation. If you feel dizzy, you open the window to have some fresh air to blow onto your face. The fresh air method could stop the car sickness and dizziness and avoid vomiting.

CHAPTER 16

Slam Your Fat Belly

Method 1: Exercise

Tighten your belly muscle with a simple exercise.

a)   Stand straight and hold the chair's high back. Look forward far and keep your neck straight.

b)   Move your *right* leg backward as far as you can until you feel your belly muscle tightening from the leg movement. Repeat this ten times.

c)   Move your *left* leg backward as far as you can until you feel your belly muscle tightening from the leg movement. Repeat this ten times.

Do this exercise whenever you have a chance at office and at home.

Method 2: Ginger Treatment on Belly Button

In the market, there are so many kinds of weight loss products now. You can select a few of them to try based on your personal situation.

The most common fat person is growing extra fat everywhere on the body. We usually consider it caused by overeating or the habit of consuming too much fatty meat in each meal.

In this book, I share a traditional herbal method to slam the fat belly caused by heavy moisture (called *shiqi* in Chinese medicine). Some people get a big fat belly by drinking too much beer. Some people get a big fat belly by eating a big meal with a lot of meat late night from 10:00 p.m. to 12:00 a.m. before sleeping.

What is shiqi? *Shiqi* is a condition where there is water retention/"dampness" in the body from excessive accumulation of moisture and not having it discharged in time. Years of fatigue can lead to decreased metabolism and bad lifestyle habits. When the weather is hot, the body becomes hot and damp, and when the weather is cold, it becomes cold and damp. Everyone's situation is different, so you need a targeted therapy guided by Chinese herb doctors.

To completely remove the extra moisture in the body, people must start by treating the spleen and stomach. Sometimes it is difficult to dispel using common methods. In that case, you need to do targeted body recovery.

First, we need to know what kind of situation caused the belly to be bigger than other parts of our body. For example, if the belly is growing so much fat that it's bigger than the arms and legs, it might be a physical sickness—shiqi.

Shiqi could also cause eczema or a fungal infection on your hands or feet. When it is on the feet, it's called athlete's foot. I will write these two common skin issues' treatment methods in a separate chapter.

Second, I suggest you begin adjusting your lifestyle. Have a balanced work and rest schedule to rest well each night. Do not stay up late. Get up at 5:00 a.m. or 6:00 a.m. and sleep before 10:00 p.m. Do some exercises each day to give the body a good restorative environment. Take a nap after lunch if needed.

Eat some food that is good for the spleen and for clearing up the dampness (with respect to diet). It is particularly important to avoid eating a big meal with a lot of meat after 10:00 p.m. and right before sleeping at night.

Third, I will introduce to you a good method that uses a natural plant—ginger—to ensure safety and no harm on the body. This method has been proven to help people who have had many years of heat and dampness coexisting accompanied by various concurrent symptoms like insomnia, bad breath, acne, bad stomach, car sickness, etc.

1.   Cut one piece of fresh ginger into small pieces.
2.   Dip a cotton swab in a little 70 percent isopropyl alcohol to gently clean your belly button.
3.   Put some small ginger pieces on the belly button.
4.   Add one drop of vinegar on top of the ginger pieces at the belly button.
5.   Tape the ginger to the belly button with a large bandage.
6.   *Optional:* For people who want to lose more fat on the belly, you can use a new and clean plastic bag (large 33 gal. size) around your belly (with the fresh ginger pieces at the belly button) tightly before sleeping. It might make some sweat come out from the belly. Clean it out with warm water when you wake up.

Continue doing this for a month. You will feel that the ginger method restored the metabolism of your spleen and stomach so that moisture will not relapse. The symptoms of insomnia, halitosis, acne, obesity, sweating, chills, etc. will completely disappear or at least visibly improve, depending on each person's body condition.

Method 3: Ginger, Black Pepper, and Dried Red Dates Juice

Use ginger, black pepper, and red dates as food medicine to help discharge the extra wet and fatty from eating fatty foods that caused the fat belly.

Materials needed: six pieces of dates, 3g of black pepper, a large piece of ginger

Preparation: Cut the ginger into small pieces. Clean the dates. See picture below.

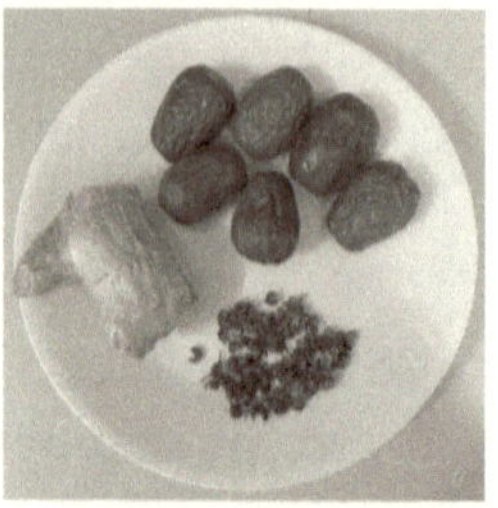

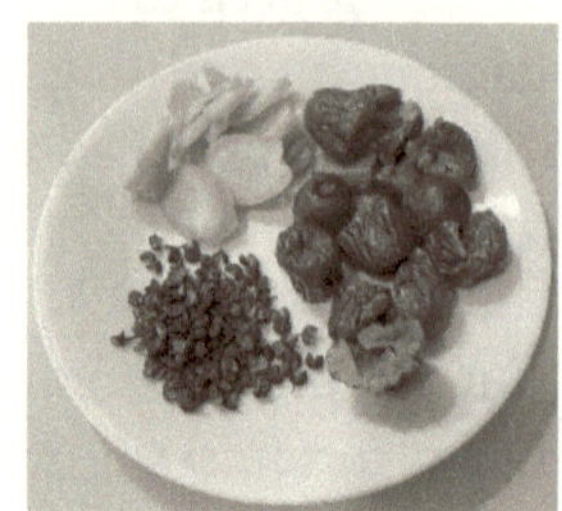

Use a pot to cook the ginger and dried red dates with a full bowel of water. When the water is boiled, turn the stove on low/medium heat to cook the ginger and dates together for fifteen minutes. You can add some brown sugar for better taste. Eat the dates and ginger. Drink the juice. Take this food medicine daily for three days, when you feel that you need it. Ginger can make you feel warm.

Note: Do not add sugar for diabetes patient.

Method 4: Apple and Dates Juice

Use apple and red dates as food medicine to help discharge the extra wet and fatty from eating fatty foods that caused the fat belly.

Materials needed: six pieces of dates, an apple, black pepper is optional to add or not add. Apple can slam the fat belly.

Preparation: Cut the apple into small pieces. Clean the dates. See picture below.

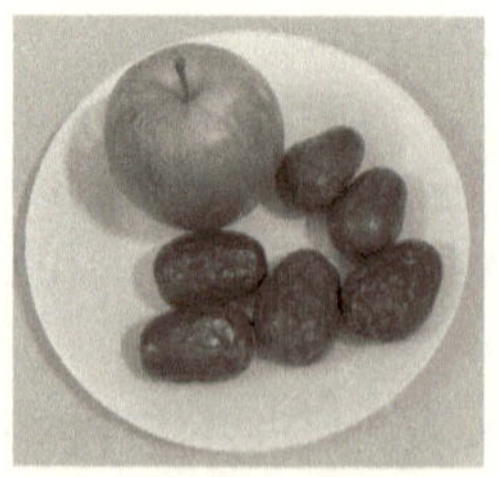

Apple and dates

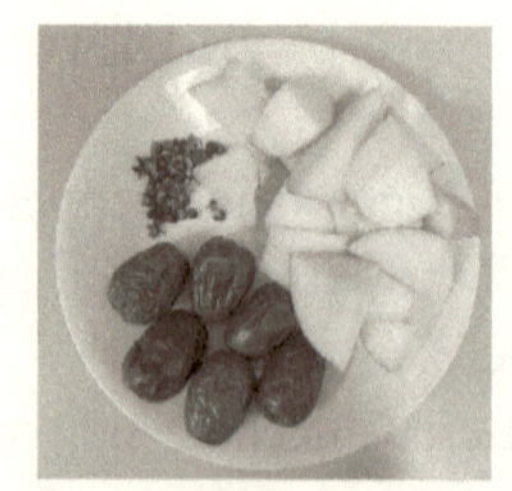

Cut apple to small pieces

Use a pot to cook the apple pieces and dried red dates with a full bowel of water. When the water is boiled, turn the stove on low/medium heat to cook the apple and dates together for fifteen minutes. You can add some brown sugar for better taste. Eat the dates and apple. Drink the juice. Take this food medicine daily for three days when you feel that you need it.

CHAPTER 17

Body Cramp Treatment

When we say "body cramp," we usually mean leg cramp, arm cramp, and hand cramp. The main cause of cramps is a lack of movement for a long time; there is a sudden increase momentum, causing strain on the muscle (e.g., the gastrocnemius muscle on the leg) or fascia inflammation. There is abnormal discharge, and the phenomenon of muscle twitching appears.

Personally, I have experienced leg cramps many times myself in my teenage years when I swam two to three extra hours. Sometimes my leg or foot cramped in that situation. Here is the urgent care I learned from my parents: Do not try to bend the leg or foot. Do not touch it. Let your body relax. After five to ten minutes of relaxing, my leg and foot started becoming soft and could move freely again, which meant it was back to normal. However, it was time for me to stop the swimming activity.

These are some treatment recommendations for cramps:

a) Maintain adequate rest and reduce leg weight-bearing activities when the body cramp happens.

b) To avoid cramps, exercise your body daily to build up strong muscles on your arms and legs. Gradually increase exercise or the amount of activity under your coach's advice. Do a good amount of warm-up activities before a big event.

c)   Apply hot compress. Massage and physiotherapy can also be used to promote blood circulation.

d)   Take an appropriate amount of calcium supplements.

If the pain persists for a long time, you need to go to the orthopedic department of the hospital for further examination and treatment.

CHAPTER 18

Treatment for Athlete's Foot

Before sleeping at night, soak your feet into warm salt water for ten minutes. Dry your feet with a clean dry towel, then sprinkle some baby powder to treat the wetness between the toes. Do it daily.

Athlete's foot is a skin problem on the feet and can be transferred through shoes. For example, if you wear someone else's shoe and they have athlete's foot, you could get the same problem from the dirty shoe. Do not wear your friend's shoe when you know they have athlete's foot.

You need to treat the stinky shoe. Athlete's foot can make their shoes stinky. Mash two mothballs into powder then sprinkle the powder into each shoe. Mothballs not only kill clothes moths and their eggs and larvae but also remove the stinky smell in the shoe.

CHAPTER 19

Sauna Bath: Benefits and Caution

A sauna is also known as a Finnish bath because the sauna originated in Finland and dates back to more than two thousand years. It is a process of physical therapy using steam in an enclosed room. The temperature in the sauna can reach up to and above 60 °C. It uses steam produced from pouring cold water on hot rocks to wash the body. This makes the blood vessels repeatedly dilate and contract and can enhance hemal elasticity. It can, therefore, prevent hemal sclerosis.

Saunas can speed up blood circulation to make the muscles of each part of the body completely relax. It can eliminate fatigue, restore physical strength, and feeling mentally energized. Plus, using the sauna has certain effects on rheumatism, arthritis, back pain, asthma, bronchitis, neurasthenia, etc. In addition, the traditional sauna has an inherent health care effect. It is a kind of enjoyment and leisure activity and is a treat for the overworked body of working-class people.

High-temperature environments have an effect on our skin-deep internal heat; there is a systemic capillary expansion, causing the body to sweat much more than when doing ordinary activities at other times. This carefree sweating is conducive to the discharge of various garbage and toxins inside the body and is also conducive to the elimination of diseases such as skin problems.

In the wintertime at the very cold northern part of the Earth, temperatures could go down to -10 °C. It is understandable that people created the sauna to survive the cold weather.

I remember that some students said, "The cold is getting into my bones in the late winter night," while they came back home from studying and research activities at the university. This was when I was living in the northern part of the United States. We shared a method of taking *hot* baths to remove the cold from body.

I had enjoyed ice fishing in the wintertime when the lake was frozen over. We drilled a hole about twelve inches wide and caught many fish there. Sometimes my body felt so cold during the fishing activity that we had to go back home early. I found a good way to recover from the cold, and that uses the concept of the sauna.

First, I rinse my body with warm water for a few minutes while I clean the bathtub. Then I soak my body in *hot* water that is about 40 °C—a temperature my body can tolerate—for about thirty minutes and finish the bath with soap. I then rinse my body with warm water for a minute before coming out.

This is an easy way to treat *cold* away from the body at home when there is no sauna facility near your residential community.

Caution: Medical experts have warned that frequent visits to the sauna could be a major cause of male infertility due to the high temperature.

For senior people who have heart diseases, they must consult with a doctor before doing sauna.

CHAPTER 20

Diabetes Care and Sugar Control in Meals

Based on medical research and study, diabetes is related to genetics and environmental factors. It should be noted that the genetic background only gives individuals a certain degree of susceptibility to diabetes; it's not enough to cause the disease.

Diabetes is generally caused by the overall effect of multiple genetic abnormalities under the action of environmental factors—eating habits, lifestyles, lack of daily exercising, etc.

Eating sugar will not lead to diabetes, but if you eat too much sugar for a long time, it will increase the burden of the pancreas and induce obesity, which is a risk factor that leads to the occurrence of diabetes.

To avoid the threat of diabetes, we must eat a balanced diet and maintain a healthy lifestyle.

In healthy individuals, if the pancreas is functioning properly, when food enters the body, sugar is broken down into glucose. Glucose then passes into the bloodstream and becomes blood sugar. Elevated blood sugar levels stimulate the beta cells in the pancreas to secrete insulin, which lowers blood sugar levels and keeps glucose levels in the blood within the normal range.

Reference ranges: Normal fasting condition blood glucose is 3.9–6.1 mmol/L. Normal postprandial blood glucose is 7.8–11.1 mmol/L

Whether the blood glucose is high or not depends on whether the blood glucose is measured on an empty stomach or after a meal. The target blood glucose levels for diabetic patients needs to be based on the patient's condition, complications caused by diabetes, as well as their age so as to establish the most suitable target level of blood glucose.

For some people who have lived with bad lifestyle habits for years (either one of these or a combination of the following: alcohol, obesity, overeating, loving sweets, etc.), these habits will increase the burden on the body's regulation of blood sugar.

Here are things you can do to manage the blood sugar and keep it within the normal ranges:

a)   Eat fruits that contain less sugar such as apple, orange, pear, etc. Eat a variety of fruit each week.
b)   Use less oil in dishes. Cook healthier food by steaming instead of using oil to fry.
c)   Fish and shrimp contain less fat than pork and beef. Therefore, eating less pork and beef is good for health.

What kind of food is good for managing diabetes? Green leafy vegetables, corn, buckwheat, wheat bran, soybeans, black beans, bitter melon, etc. have low glycemic effect and rich dietary fiber; these have certain effects on blood glucose control.

CHAPTER 21

Balanced Body Energy
for Mind Wellness

Physical wellness is a combination of living well with the daily schedule of study well (for students) / working well (for adults), eating three meals (breakfast, lunch, and dinner) on time, and resting well at night.

Physical wellness brings the family happiness. Trust God; if there is anything that you cannot resolve, God can. Just let God take care of it for you.

Seventeen years ago, when my right hand was broken due to a fall on the ground at Skateland, I thought positively that my hand is broken, so my daughter's hands and legs are saved. Because she asked me to take her to play at the four-wheel shoe Skating Land every weekend.

I could not take care my two children aged ten and six at home anymore, so I prayed to God, asking him to take care of them for me and to make them useful and helpful. God listened and helped. Now they both have completed their college education and are working in jobs.

According to a recent study by researchers, religious practice may be beneficial to physical and mental health. Researchers at Duke University Medical Center in the United States conducted a series of studies to explore the relationship between religion and human health. The result is promisingly good and healthy.

These are what the Bible teaches:

a)   God cares about you personally (Peter 5:7).
b)   God's personal name is Jehovah (Psalm 83:18).
c)   Jehovah invites you to draw close to him (James 4:8).
d)   Jehovah is loving, kind, and merciful (Exodus 34:6; 1 John 4:8, 16).

The three major religions in the world are Buddhism, Christianity, and Islam. They all believe in God.

The founder of Buddhism is Buddha. His original name is Sakyamunī, which means "who fully realize the truth." He gained enlightenment under the bodhi tree at age thirty-five in China. He was born and named Siddhartha Gautama and was the crown prince of Kapilavastu in Nepal, India. He founded the Buddhism in the sixth and fifth century BC. He told his followers that he is God's servant.

The founder of Christianity is Jesus. According to the Bible, the Virgin Mary was conceived by the Holy Spirit and gave birth to Jesus in Bethlehem. He started preaching at the age of thirty. Jesus told his followers that he is the son of God. Jesus died on the cross to save people on earth.

The founder of Islam is Muhammad. The followers are called Muslims. Muhammad was born in a noble family (570–632), but his father passed away before he was born while his mother passed away when he was six. He was raised by his granduncle and uncle. Muhammad of Mecca on the Arabian Peninsula, introduced Islam from West Asia and the middle East to the world in the AD seventh century.

God is real. God wants the earth filled with healthy people. Please see the reference picture below from the book *What Does the Bible Really Teach?*

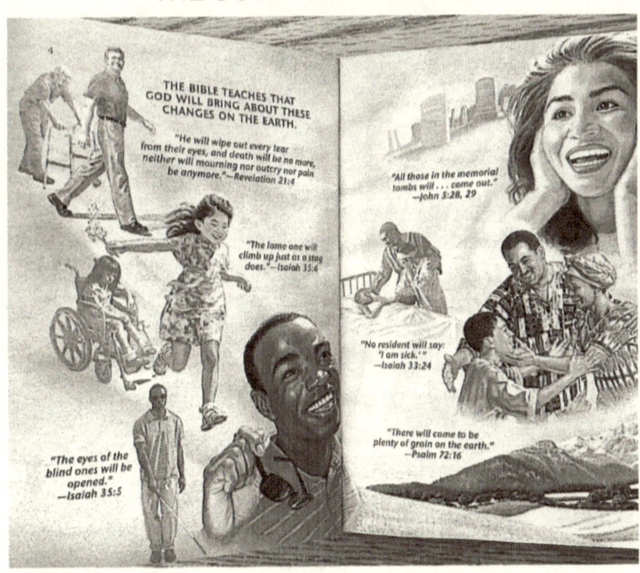

I work for God. I work on projects that contribute toward the fulfillment of God's plan to help people become healthier and happier.

So many times I heard people say, "The medical bill is so high. We can't afford it" or "We may go bankrupt from the medical expenses." Some people say, "We have to take painkiller drugs every day because my body is hurting," "I am so tired that I have to drink three cups of coffee to keep me awake," or "I am so tired, and I have to smoke to reenergize again." It all means that they need good rest to recover their bodies.

Some drugs can temporarily energize people, but after certain time, it makes people even more tired. It makes people attached to the drug again and again.

Some people increase their dosages of painkiller drugs. They eventually die from overdose.

Some people increase their dosages of energizing drugs. Their health becomes damaged. The drug can cause people depression, based on medical research and study.

No medicine can make people strong. Medicine is for healing sickness. All medicine has some side effects, so we must take medicine under a doctor's guidance.

People become stronger and stronger through work. Athletes build up their muscles and skills through years of training day by day.

This book, *How to Stay Healthy During/After COVID-19 Pandemic?*, has the same purpose of keeping people healthy; it provides some information on herbs and methods for using them that were used in the ancient years when treating some sicknesses and symptoms as they began to manifest. They are affordable/low-cost and doable at home to help people become healthier and happier! Balance your body's energy through healthy lifestyle habits and scheduling time for mind wellness too.

CHAPTER 22

Goal-Setting for Your Career Success

A healthy body starts with a healthy mind. Goal-setting is great for adults and students. Write down the weekly and monthly goals you want to accomplish in your career. Study while following a daily exercise plan and schedule to maintain a healthy body. From this, you have a good, healthy body to accomplish your goals every day.

Setting a long-term goal for the year is also important for achieving your career goal. Once you have the year's goal set, you will be able to look at it from your current point of view to see how much work you need to do to accomplish the goal. This way, you can schedule and manage your daily life more efficiently.

In life, we get some unexpected situations that might delay our schedule to reach the goal. We must forgive ourselves as we often forgive others. My advice is to treat yourself to a nice meal. Rest well to recover your body's energy first to overcome the unexpected situation. Plan a day or a week to catch up with some workload so you will feel better again.

Life has ups and downs. Stay modest in the ups and keep self-respect in the downs. Trust God and know that everything will come to pass. The important thing is to learn from it. Do better soon.

In the career competition, other people cannot fail you. Only you can fail yourself. Make sure your goal-setting is in good faith. Get back to work again after recharging your body's energy through resting, massaging, and love. Love is the cure and answer for many problems in one's personal life. Love has healing power! When our hearts are filled with love, there is no space for problems.

A career success often takes more time than just working from 9:00 a.m. to 5:00 p.m. Loving what you do and doing what you love is the key to success in your career. Every professional person can tell you that they have put much of their spare time into working to build their career. That is why people say, "Making your habit into your business is the best way to success." It's because your habit is what you love to do, even you don't get paid for doing it. It means you work for yourself to make yourself happy instead of working for others for money.

Telling yourself to "just do it" is a powerful way to accomplish your career goal. You forget the hours and labor. All your focus is on getting it done. In fact, you will be rewarded for the long term in life after you accomplish your career goal.

A car needs a good maintenance to keep running well. The human body also needs good care and health maintenance to stay away from sickness. Whenever you feel a little symptom or that you do not feel well, try some of those methods in this handbook to stay healthy and strong.

ABOUT THE AUTHOR

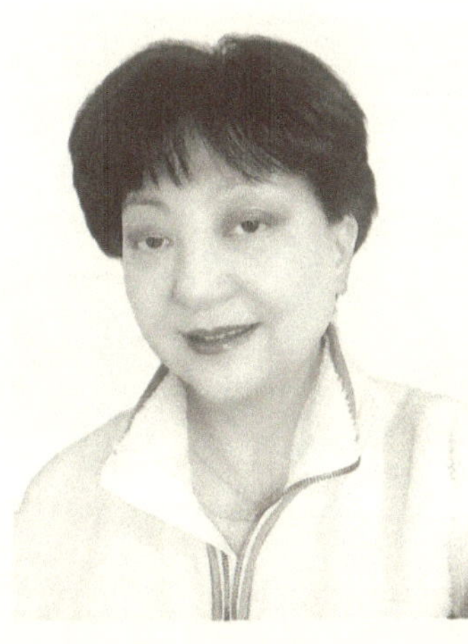

The author's name is Jing Carter-Lu (previously known as Jing Lu). She's an entrepreneur and inventor.

She was homeschooled in medicine in her childhood because her father was a doctor and one of the managers who runs a medicine and medical equipment company.

She worked for their local city's Industry and Commerce Business Administration Bureau for six years since she was twenty-one years old. She earned the scholarship at her workplace to complete her college education, in which she majored in industry and commerce administration. She teamed up with their director to compile and publish two law books: *Economic Laws Collection* and *Industrial and Commercial Administration Laws and Regulations Compilation*.

She came to the United States in 1990. She worked for Weill Medical College of Cornell University for seven years as a research technician, where she received the honor of her name being listed as one of the authors in seven scientific research papers and two patents.

She started her first company—Healthier & Happier, Inc.—in July 2003. They provided import and export services and B2B services.

She wrote a patent in 2009 and filed continue-in-part patent application in 2012 for improving indoor air quality that had been granted in May 2016 by the USPTO with US Utility Patent No. 9,352,259 and titled "System, Method, and Devices for Air

Filtration." Based on her patent, she created the product lines and established a manufacturing company: Eco-safe Air Filters Manufacturing Company in 2015.

Her goal in life and in business/work is to contribute benefits to help people become *healthier and happier*.